SIRTFOOD DIET RECIPES

Easy And Delicious Recipes To Activate Your Skinny Gene

GLENDA HAMILTON

TABLE OF CONTENTS

Introduction

Sirtfoods are a group of nutrient-rich foods that were recently discovered and are very useful for persons willing to lose weight. Sirtuins are much considered compared to other fasting-diet foods since they do not show critical disadvantages like muscle loss, irritability, and hunger—Diet founder's work by activating a specific type of proteins called sirtuins. Sirtuins work by protecting body cells from dying. Sirtuins are also able to burn fats at a high rate, hence boosting metabolism. The main sirtfoods available are apples, dark chocolate, green tea, kale, blueberries, red wine, capers, turmeric, citrus fruits, and parsley.

In 2003, a landmark study on nutrition and diets found that Resveratrol, a compound found in grape skin and red wine, has the capability of increasing the lifespan of yeast significantly. Also, the same compound was found to restrict calories from building up in the body. Over the years, more studies have been conducted on Resveratrol, and these studies have shown that it has a positive effect on extending life in honeybees, fish, worms, and flies. In humans, this magic compound was discovered to have a significant impact on protecting bod-

1

ies against the harsh effects of high-sugar, high-fat, and high-calories on the human body.

This landmark discovery made the abundant resveratrol compound in red wine to make red wine be considered as the original sirtfood ever discovered. The health benefits of red wine on the body has remarkable health benefits which make it a wonder drink, being sort by people all over so that they can lose their weight. The discovery of Resveratrol paved the way for more in-depth research on food that can have significant impacts on the human body. Researchers began the work of looking into different compounds in different foods that can have the ability to activate sirtuin genes. A few years later, tens of compounds were discovered to have a similar effect, like Resveratrol.

Red wine is the original Sirtfood discovered, which allowed researchers to look more into the plant. It was later found that they would maximize the effect of sirtuin genes in the body as well as the absorption of critical nutrients in the body. Some of the other compounds discovered in red wine included myricetin, piceatannol, and epicatechin. Each of these compounds had a similar effect in activating sirtuin genes as the coordination was perfect. Other vital foods in the Sirt food diet, after analysis, were found to have related or compounds with a similar effect.

A Sirt food diet is highly recommended, especially for individuals who require a high mineral and vitamin intake in their bodies. One thing about sirtfoods is that they are quite restrictive when it comes to calories and the amount of food you take. This, therefore, may deem not so pleasant for a person who likes to eat anything they like at any time. Sirtfoods are mainly for people who want to lose weight. Such individuals would, therefore, not feel the pinch of the diet since they are after a particular goal.

Despite the myriad health benefits that sirtfoods pose, there a group of people that are advised not to take sirtfoods. One group of people in this category is people with prevailing health conditions like diabetes. Medical experts argue that stringent diets like the Sirt food diet may deprive the body of essential sugars, which may worsen the status of a diabetic patient. Also, people under medication due to various body issues may have complications if they settle to the Sirt food diet. However, if the diet is complemented with other foods, the benefits are immeasurable. Apart from the few exempted individuals, sirtfoods are recommended for anyone who seeks to stay in shape.

Chapter 1: Sirtfood Ingredients

THE BEST 20 SIRTFOODS

Now that you know all about Sirtfoods, why they're so good, and what it takes to build a successful diet that will produce lasting results, it's time to get started.

ARUGULA

In US food culture, Arugula (also known as rocket, rucola, arugula, and roquette) definitely has a colorful past. A pungent green salad leaf with a distinctive peppery taste, it rapidly ascended from humble origins as the basis of many Mediterranean peasant dishes to become a symbol of food snobbery in the United States, also contributing to the coining of the word arugula!

BUCKWHEAT

Buckwheat was one of Japan's earliest domesticated crops, and the story goes that when Buddhist monks made long mountain trips, all they would bring was a cooking pot and buckwheat bag for food. Buckwheat is so nutritious that this was all they wanted, and it kept them up for weeks. We're big fans of buckwheat too. Second, since it is one of a sirtuin activator's best-known sources named rutin. But also, because it has benefits as a cover crop, improving soil quality and suppressing weed growth, making it a fantastic crop for sustainable and environmentally friendly agriculture.

CAPERS

If you're not so familiar with capers, we're talking about those salty, dark green, pellet-like stuff you might only have had an opportunity to see on top of a pizza. But certainly, they are one of the most undervalued and neglected foods out there. Intriguingly, they are, in fact, the caper bush's owner buds, which grow abundantly in the Mediterranean before being picked and preserved by hand.

CELERY

For centuries, Celery has been around and revered—with leaves found to adorn the remains of the Egyptian pharaoh Tutankhamun who died around 1323 BCE. Early strains were very bitter, and celery was commonly considered a medicinal plant, particularly for washing and detoxification to prevent disease. The fact that liver, kidney, and gut safety are among the multitude of promising benefits that science is now demonstrating is especially important.

CHILIES

Chili has been an integral part of the gastronomic experience world-wide for thousands of years. At one point, we would be so enamored of it; it's baffling. Its pungent fire, caused by a substance called capsaicin in chilies, is designed as a plant defence mechanism to cause pain and dissuade predators from feasting on it, and we appreciate that. The food and our infatuation with it are almost magical.

COCOA

We saw the impressive health benefits of cocoa on pages 59–60, so it's no surprise to hear that cocoa was considered a sacred food for ancient civilizations like the Aztecs and Mayans, and was generally reserved for the wealthy and the warriors, served at feasts to obtain allegiance and obligation. Indeed, there was such high regard for the cocoa bean that it was even used as a form of currency. It was usually served as a frothy beverage back then. But what could be a more delicious way to get our dietary quota of cacao than by chocolate?

COFFEE

What's all that about Sirtfood coffee? We're listening to you. We can assure you that there is no typo. Gone are the days when a twinge of remorse had to balance our enjoyment of coffee. Work is unambiguous: coffee is a bona de alimentation. In reality, it is a true treasure trove of fantastic nutrients that trigger Sirtuin. And with more than half of Americans drinking coffee every day (to the tune of $40 billion a year!), coffee boasts the accolade of being America's number one source of polyphenols.

EXTRA VIRGIN OLIVE OIL

Olive oil is a traditional Mediterranean diet's most renowned food. The olive tree is among the world's oldest-known cultivated plants, also known as the "immortal tree." And since people started squeezing olives in stone mortars to gather them, the oil has been worshipped, almost 7,000 years ago. Hippocrates quoted it as a cure-all; now, a few centuries, modern science firms its wonderful wellbeing benefits un-mistakably.

GARLIC

For thousands of years, garlic has been considered as one of the wonder foods of nature, with healing and rejuvenating properties. Egyptians fed pyramid crews with garlic to enhance their immunity, avoid various diseases, and strengthen their performance through their ability to prevent fatigue. Garlic is a potent natural antibiotic and antifungal that is sometimes used to help cure ulcers in the stomach. By promoting the elimination of waste products from the body, it can activate the lymphatic system to "detox" So besides being investigated for fat loss, it also packs a potent heart health punch, lowering cholesterol by around 10 percent so reducing blood pressure by 5 to 7 percent, as well as reducing blood and blood sugar stickiness.

GREEN TEA (ESPECIALLY MATCHA)

Green tea, the Orient's toast and becoming increasingly popular in the West, will be familiar to many. As well as the growing awareness of its health benefits, green tea consumption is linked to less cancer, heart disease, diabetes, and osteoporosis. The reason it is thought that green tea is so good for us is mainly due to its rich content of a group of powerful plant compounds called catechins, the star of the show being a specific form of sirtuin-activating catechin known as epigallocatechin gallate (EGCG).

KALE

You can never go wrong with some leafy greens, and this is applicable for kale as well. Kale has become very popular and appreciated over the last few years by both nutritionists and consumers, and they have all the reasons to like and appreciate it. This leafy green is among the best sources of kaempferol and quercetin, nutrients capable of triggering sirtuins. Therefore, kale should not be missing from your sirtfood diet, and you can easily make your own juices using it. Another great fact about kale is that it is not something exotic, a very rare vegetable available on a remote tropical island. This leafy green can be grown locally, so it is very accessible and affordable.

MEDJOOL DATES

It may come as a surprise to include Medjool dates in a list of foods that stimulate weight loss and promote health—especially when we tell you that Medjool dates contain a whopping 66 percent sugar. Sugar doesn't have any sirtuin-activating properties at all; instead, it has well-established links to obesity, heart disease, and diabetes—just the opposite of what we're looking to achieve.

PARSLEY

Parsley is a gastronomic conundrum. It so often appears in recipes, yet so often it's the green token man. At best, we serve a couple of chopped sprigs and tossed as an afterthought on a meal, at worst a solitary sprig for decorative purposes only. Either way, there on the plate, it is often still languishing long after we've eaten finish. This culinary style derives from its common use in ancient Rome as a garnish for eating after meals in order to restore oxygen, rather than being part of the meal itself. And what a shame, because parsley is a fantastic food that packs a vivid and refreshing flavor that is a character filled with.

RED ENDIVE

The endive is a relatively new kid on the block, as far as vegetables go. Legend has it that a Belgian farmer found endive in 1830, by mistake. The farmer stored chicory roots in his cellar, and then used them as a form of coffee substitute, only to forget them. Upon his return, he discovered that white leaves had sprouted, which he considered being soft, crunchy, and very tasty upon degustation. Endive is now grown all over the world, including the USA, and earns its Sirtfood badge thanks to its outstanding sirtuin activator luteolin material. And besides the well-established sirtuin-activating benefits, luteolin intake has become a promising approach to therapy to improve sociability in autistic children.

RED ONIONS

Red Onions have been a dietary staple from the time of our prehistoric ancestors, being one of the first crops to be grown, around 5,000 years ago. With such a long history of use and such strong health-giving properties, many cultures that came before us have revered onions. They were held especially by the Egyptians as objects of worship, regarding their circle-within-a-circle structure as symbolic of eternal life. And the Greeks believed that onions made athletes stronger. Athletes will eat their way through large quantities of onions before the Olympic Games, including consuming the juice! It's an amazing testament to how important ancient dietary knowledge can be when we remember that onions deserve their top twenty Sirtfood status because they're chock-full of the sirtuin-activating compound quercetin—the very compound that the sports science world has recently started aggressively researching and promoting to boost sports performance.

RED WINE

Any list of the top twenty Sirtfoods will not be complete without red wine, the original Sirtfood, being included. The French phenomenon made headlines in the early 1990s, with it being discovered that despite the French appearing to do something wrong when it came to health (smoking, lack of exercise, and rich food consumption), they had lower death rates from heart disease than countries like the United States. Doctors suggested the explanation for this was the copious amount of red wine drank.

SOY

Soy products have a long history as an important part of the diet of many countries in Asia-Paci, such as China, Japan, and Korea. After observing that high soy-consuming countries had significantly lower levels of certain cancers, particularly breast and prostate, researchers first turned on to soy. This is believed to be due to a special group of polyphenols in soybeans known as isoflavones, which can favorably affect how estrogen functions in the body, like daidzein formononetin sirtuin-activators. Soy product intake has also been related to a decrease in the incidence or severity of a number of conditions such as cardiovascular disease, effects of menopause, and bone loss.

STRAWBERRIES

In recent years, Strawberries Fruit has been increasingly vilified, getting a bad rap in the rising fervor against sugar. Luckily, such a malignant image couldn't be more undeserved for berry-lovers. While all the berries are powerhouses of nutrition, strawberries gain their top twenty Sirtfood status due to their sirtuin activator set in abundance. And now studies support daily eating strawberries to encourage healthy aging, keeping off Alzheimer's, obesity, diabetes, heart disease, and osteoporosis. As for their sugar content, a pure teaspoon of sugar per 3/2 ounces is very small.

TURMERIC

Turmeric, a cousin of ginger, is the latest kid in food trends on the block with Google calling it the 2015 ingredient "breakout star." While we are only turning to it nowhere in the West, it has been valued for thousands of years in Asia, for both culinary and medical reasons. Incredibly, India is generating almost the entire world's turmeric supply, eating 80 percent of it itself. Before Indian weddings, there is a ritual where the turmeric paste is applied as a skin beauty treatment to the bride and groom, but also to symbolize the warding off evil.

WALNUTS

According to the NuVal system, walnuts lead the way as the number one nut for health, which ranks foods according to how safe they are and has been endorsed by the American College of Preventive Medicine. But what really makes walnuts stand out for us is how they stand out against conventional thinking: they are high in fat and calories, yet well-established for weight reduction and the risk of metabolic diseases such as cardiovascular disease and diabetes being reduced. That is the strength of triggering the Sirtuin.

MORE SIRTFOODS FOR YOUR RECIPES

SEAFOOD

Seafood means fish like sardines, mackerel, and wild salmon. It's also a good idea to add some shrimp, tuna, mussels, and crab into your diet. This is going to be a tad expensive, but worth it in the long run. What's the common denominator in all these food items? The secret is omega-3 fatty acids, which are credited for lots of health benefits. You want to add food rich in omega-3 fatty acids to your diet.

LOW-CARB VEGETABLES

The Vegetable Choices Should be limited to those with low carbohydrate counts. Pack up your cart with items like spinach, eggplant, arugula, broccoli, and cauliflower. You can also put in bell peppers, cabbage, celery, kale, Brussels sprouts, mushrooms, zucchini, and fennel.

So, what's in them? Well, aside from the fact that they're low carb, these vegetables also contain loads of fiber, which makes digestion easier. Of course, there's also the presence of vitamins, minerals, antioxidants, and various other nutrients that you need for day-to-day life. Which ones should you avoid? Steer clear of the starch-packed vegetables like carrots, turnips, and beets. As a rule, you go for the plants that are green and leafy.

FRUITS LOW IN SUGAR

During an episode of sugar-craving, it's usually a good idea to pick low-sugar fruit items. Believe it or not, there are lots of those in the market! Just make sure to stock up on any of these: avocado, blackberries, raspberries, strawberries, blueberries, lime, lemon, and coconut. Also, note that tomatoes are fruits too, so feel free to make side dishes or dips with loads of vegetables! Keep in mind that these fruits should be eaten fresh and not out of a can. However, if you do eat them raw off the box, take a good look at the nutritional information at the back of the packaging. Avocadoes are particularly popular for those practicing the Sirtfoods Diet because they contain LOTS of the right kind of fat.

MEAT AND EGGS

While some diets will tell you to skip the meat, the Sirtfood Diet encourages its consumption. Chicken is packed with protein that will feed your muscles and give you a consistent source of energy throughout the day. It's a slow but sure burn when you eat protein as opposed to carbohydrates, which are burned faster and therefore stored faster if you don't use them immediately.

But what kind of meat should you be eating? There's chicken, beef, pork, venison, turkey, and lamb. Keep in mind that quality plays a huge role here—you should be eating grass-fed organic beef or organic poultry if you want to make the most out of this food variety. The nuclear option lets you limit the possibility of ingesting toxins in your body due to the production process of these products. Plus, the preservation process also means there is added salt or sugar in the meat, which can throw off the whole diet.

NUTS AND SEEDS

The nuts and seeds you should add to your cart include chia seeds, brazil nuts, macadamia nuts, flaxseed, walnuts, hemp seeds, pecans, sesame seeds, almonds, hazelnut, and pumpkin seeds. They also contain lots of protein and very little sugar, so they're great if you have the munchies. They're the ideal snack because they're quick, easy, and will keep you full. They're high in calories, though, which is why lots of people steer clear of them.

DAIRY PRODUCTS

Some people in their 50 already have a hard time processing dairy products, but for those who don't, you can happily add many of these to your diet. Make sure to consume sufficient amounts of cheese, plain Greek yogurt, cream butter, and cottage cheese. These dairy products are packed with calcium, protein, and a healthy kind of fat.

COFFEE AND TEA

The good news is that you don't have to skip coffee if you're going on a Sirtfoods Diet. The bad news is that you can't go to Starbucks anymore and order their blended coffee choices. Instead, beverages would be limited to unsweetened tea or unsweetened coffee to keep sugar consumption low option for organic coffee and tea products to make the most out of these powerful antioxidants.

DARK CHOCOLATE

Yes—chocolate is still on the menu, but it is limited to just dark chocolate. Technically, this means eating chocolate that is 70 percent cacao, which would make the taste a bit bitter.

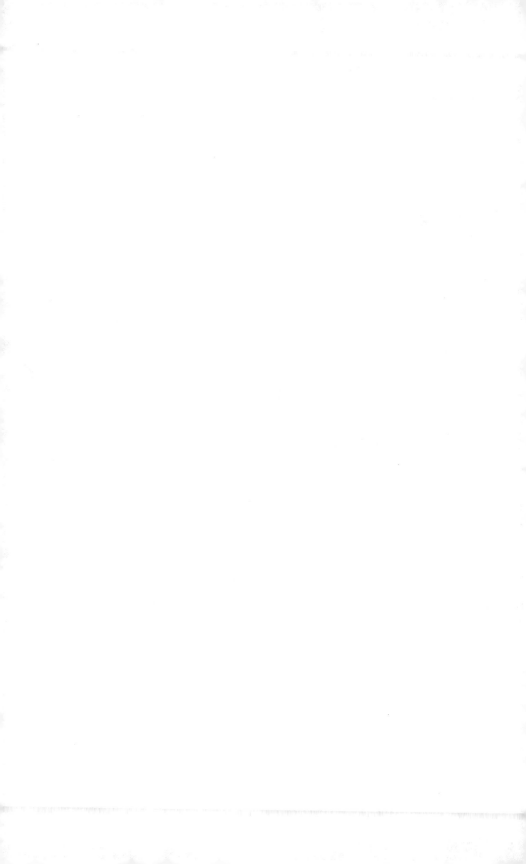

Chapter 2: Sirtfood Green Juice Collection

GREEN JUICE

Preparation Time: 10 minutes
Cooking Time: 0 minutes
Servings: 2

INGREDIENTS:

- 75g Kale
- 30g Rocket
- 5g Flat-leaf parsley
- 5g Lovage leaves
- 150g Celery
- ½ a green apple
- Juice of ½ a lemon
- ½ level tsp. Matcha

Whilst these are the official measurements, you can generally approximate the recipe as follows;

- 2 handfuls of kale
- 1 handful of rocket
- A pinch of parsley
- A pinch of lovage
- 3 large celery stalks
- ½ a green apple
- Juice of ½ a lemon
- ½ level tsp. Matcha

DIRECTIONS:

1. Using the handful measurement also helps you to adjust how you make the green juice—people with larger bodies (and larger hands) will receive slightly more of each ingredient, which should ensure that they are getting proportionally enough.

2. Start making the green juice by juicing the leafy greens and herbs—you should be aiming to produce about 50ml of liquid. Juicers vary in their ability to process the greens, so you might need multiple processing attempts to generate the juice.

3. Next add the celery and apple, juicing once more. Squeeze in the lemon juice and blend again. You should have approximately 1 cup (250ml) of juice to work with.

4. Separate the juice into two equal-sized portions. Toss in the Matcha to one portion, stirring vigorously. Matcha is only added to the morning and the midday juice as it contains noticeable amounts of caffeine and may keep you awake in the evening. After the Matcha has been absorbed, pour the two portions back together and stir.

5. Your juice is now ready. You may want to add some water, ac-

cording to your own sense of taste. There is no need to make the juice from scratch every time you want it—you can produce batches, which should stay fresh and not lose any of their value for up to 3 days, as long as you keep them chilled.

NUTRITION:

- Calories 250
- Carbs 47.9g
- Protein 5.2g

LEMONY GREEN JUICE

Preparation Time: 10 minutes
Cooking Time: 0 minutes
Servings: 2

INGREDIENTS:

- 2 large green apples, cored and sliced
- 4 cups fresh kale leaves
- 4 tablespoons fresh parsley leaves
- 1 tablespoon fresh ginger, peeled
- 1 lemon, peeled
- ½ cup filtered water
- Pinch of salt

DIRECTIONS:

1. Place all the ingredients in a blender and pulse until well combined.

2. Through a fine mesh strainer, strain the juice and transfer into 2glasses.

3. Serve immediately.

NUTRITION:

- Calories 196
- Fat 0.6g
- Carbs 47.9g
- Protein 5.2g

Matcha Green Juice

Preparation Time: 10 minutes
Cooking Time: 0 minutes
Servings: 2

INGREDIENTS:

- 5 ounces fresh kale
- 2 ounces fresh arugula
- ¼ cup fresh parsley
- 4 celery stalks
- 1green apple, cored and chopped
- 1 (1-inch) piece fresh ginger, peeled
- 1 lemon, peeled
- ½ teaspoon matcha green tea

DIRECTIONS:

1. Add all ingredients into a juicer and extract the juice according to the manufacturer's method.
2. Pour into 2 glasses and serve immediately.

NUTRITION:

- Calories 113
- Fat 0.6g
- Carbs 26.71g
- Protein 3.8g

CELERY JUICE

Preparation Time: 10 minutes
Cooking Time: 0 minutes
Servings: 2

INGREDIENTS:

- 8 celery stalks with leaves
- 2 tablespoons fresh ginger, peeled
- 1 lemon, peeled
- ½ cup filtered water
- Pinch of salt

DIRECTIONS:

1. Place all the ingredients in a blender and pulse until well combined.
2. Through a fine mesh strainer, strain the juice and transfer into 2glasses.
3. Serve immediately.

NUTRITION:

- Calories 32
- Fat 0.5g
- Carbs 6.5g
- Protein 1g

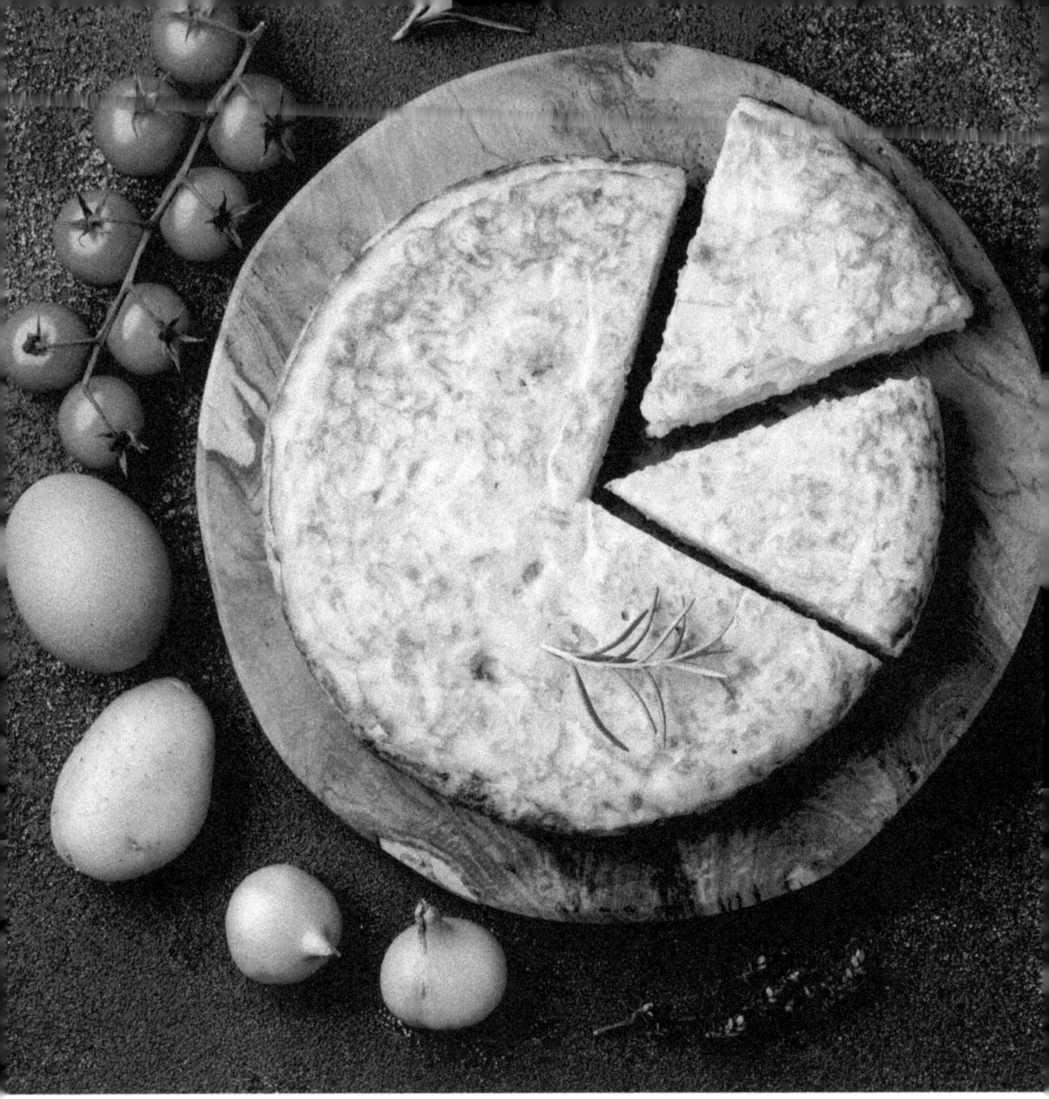

CHAPTER
03

BREAKFAST RECIPES

Chapter 3: Breakfast Recipes

CHERRY AND VANILLA PROTEIN SHAKE

Preparation Time: 5 minutes
Cooking Time: 10 minutes
Servings: 2

INGREDIENTS:

- 4 ounces cherries, destemmed
- 1 scoop vanilla protein powder
- 1 ½ cup almond milk, unsweetened

DIRECTIONS:

1. Place all the ingredients in the order into a food processor or blender, and then pulse for 1 to 2 minutes until smooth.
2. Distribute shake between two glasses and then serve.
3. Divide shake between two jars or bottles, cover with a lid, and then store the containers in the refrigerator for up to 3 days.

NUTRITION:

- Cal 193
- Fats 8g
- Protein 5.2g
- Carb 38g
- Fiber 11g

KALE SCRAMBLE

Preparation Time: 10 minutes
Cooking Time: 6 minutes
Servings: 2

INGREDIENTS:

- 4 eggs
- 1/8 teaspoon ground turmeric
- Salt and ground black pepper, to taste
- 1 tablespoon water
- 2 teaspoons olive oil
- 1 cup fresh kale, tough ribs removed and chopped

DIRECTIONS:

1. In a bowl, add the eggs, turmeric, salt, black pepper, and water and with a whisk, beat until foamy.
2. In a wok, heat the oil over medium heat.
3. Add the egg mixture and stir to combine.
4. Immediately, reduce the heat to medium-low and cook for about 1-2 minutes, stirring frequently.
5. Stir in the kale and cook for about 3-4 minutes, stirring frequently.
6. Remove from the heat and serve immediately.

NUTRITION:

- Calories 183kcal
- Fat 13.4g
- Carbs 4.3g
- Protein 12.1g

BUCKWHEAT PORRIDGE

Preparation Time: 10 minutes
Cooking Time: 15 minutes
Servings: 2

INGREDIENTS:

- 1 cup buckwheat, rinsed
- 1 cup unsweetened almond milk
- 1 cup water
- ½ teaspoon ground cinnamon
- ½ teaspoon vanilla extract
- 1-2 tablespoons raw honey
- ¼ cup fresh blueberries

DIRECTIONS:

1. In a pan, add all the ingredients (except honey and blueberries) over medium-high heat and bring to a boil.
2. Now, reduce the heat to low and simmer, covered for about 10 minutes.
3. Stir in the honey and remove from the heat.
4. Set aside, covered, for about 5 minutes.
5. With a fork, fluff the mixture, and transfer into serving bowls.
6. Top with blueberries and serve.

NUTRITION:

- Calories 358kcal
- Fat 4.7g
- Carbs 3.7g
- Protein 12g

TOMATO FRITTATA

Preparation Time: 55 minutes
Cooking Time: 20 minutes
Servings: 2

INGREDIENTS:

- 50g cheddar cheese, grated
- 75g kalamata olives, pitted and halved
- 8 cherry tomatoes, halved
- 4 large eggs
- 1 tbsp. fresh parsley, chopped
- 1 tbsp. fresh basil, chopped
- 1 tbsp. olive oil

DIRECTIONS:

1. Whisk eggs together in a large mixing bowl. Toss in the parsley, basil, olives, tomatoes and cheese, stirring thoroughly.

2. In a small skillet, heat the olive oil over high heat. Pour in the frittata mixture and cook for 5-10 minutes or set. Remove the skillet from the hob and place under the grill for 5 minutes, or until firm and set. Divide into portions and serve immediately.

NUTRITION:

- Calories 269 kcal
- Protein 9.23g
- Fat 23.76g
- Carbohydrates 5.49g

GREEN OMELET

Preparation Time: 5 minutes
Cooking Time: 35 minutes
Servings: 1

INGREDIENTS:

- 1 teaspoon of olive oil
- 1 shallot peeled and finely chopped
- 2 large eggs
- Salt
- A small handful of parsley, finely chopped
- A handful of rocket leaves about 20grams
- Freshly ground black pepper

DIRECTIONS:

1. Heat the oil in a large frying pan, over medium-low heat. Add the shallot and gently fry for about 5 minutes. Increase the heat and cook for two more minutes.

2. In a cup or bowl, whisk the eggs; evenly distribute the shallot in the pan then add in the eggs. Evenly distribute the eggs by tipping over the pan on all sides. Cook for about a minute before lifting the sides and allowing the runny eggs to move to the base of the pan.

3. Sprinkle rocket leaves and parsley on top and season with pepper and salt to taste. When the base is just starting to brown, tip it onto a plate and serve right away.

NUTRITION:

- Calories 221
- Fat 28g
- Carbohydrates 10g
- Fiber 7
- Sugar 1g

Mushroom Scramble Eggs

Preparation Time: 45 minutes
Cooking Time: 10 minutes
Servings: 2

INGREDIENTS:

- 2 eggs
- 1 tsp ground turmeric
- 1 tsp mellow curry powder
- 20g kale, generally slashed
- 1 tsp additional virgin olive oil
- ½ superior bean stews, daintily cut
- Bunch of catch mushrooms, meagerly cut
- 5g parsley, finely slashed
- *optional* Add a seed blend as a topper and some Rooster Sauce to enhance

DIRECTIONS:

1. Blend the turmeric and curry powder and include a little water until you have accomplished a light glue.

2. Steam the kale for 2-3 minutes.

3. Warmth the oil in a skillet over medium heat and fry the bean stew and mushrooms for 2 to 3 minutes until they begin to darker and mollify.

4. Include the eggs and flavor glue and cook over medium warmth at that point, add the kale and keep on cooking over medium heat for a further moment. At long last, include the parsley, blend well and serve.

NUTRITION:

- Calories 158kcal
- Protein 9.96g
- Fat 10.93g
- Carbohydrates 5.04g

SMOKED SALMON OMELET

Preparation Time: 45 minutes
Cooking Time: 15 minutes
Servings: 2

INGREDIENTS:

- 2 Medium eggs
- 100g Smoked salmon, cut
- 1/2 tsp Capers
- 10g Rocket, slashed
- 1 tsp Parsley, slashed
- 1 tsp extra virgin olive oil

DIRECTIONS:

1. Split the eggs into a bowl and whisk well. Include the salmon, tricks, rocket and parsley.

2. Warmth the olive oil in a non-stick skillet until hot, yet not smoking. Include the egg blend and, utilizing a spatula or fish cut, move the mixture around the dish until it is even. Diminish the warmth and let the Omelettes cook through. Slide the spatula around the edges and move up or crease the Omelettes fifty-fifty to serve.

NUTRITION:

- Calories 148kcal
- Protein 15.87g
- Fat 8.73g
- Carbohydrates 0.36g

SALMON & KALE OMELETTE

Preparation Time: 10 minutes
Cooking Time: 7 minutes
Servings: 4

INGREDIENTS:

- 6 eggs
- 2 tablespoons unsweetened almond milk
- Salt and ground black pepper, to taste
- 2 tablespoons olive oil
- 4 ounces smoked salmon, cut into bite-sized chunks
- 2 cup fresh kale, tough ribs removed and chopped finely
- 4 scallions, chopped finely

DIRECTIONS:

1. In a bowl, place the eggs, almond milk, salt, and black pepper, and beat well. Set aside.
2. In a non-stick wok, heat the oil over medium heat.
3. Place the egg mixture evenly and cook for about 30 seconds, without stirring.
4. Place the salmon kale and scallions on top of egg mixture evenly.
5. Now, reduce heat to low.
6. With the lid, cover the wok and cook for about 4-5 minutes, or until Omelette is done completely.
7. Uncover the wok and cook for about 1 minute.
8. Carefully, transfer the Omelette onto a serving plate and serve.

NUTRITION:

- Calories 210
- Fat 14.9g
- Carbs 5.2g
- Protein 14.8g

Moroccan Spiced Eggs

Preparation Time: 1 hour
Cooking Time: 50 minutes
Servings: 2

INGREDIENTS:

- 1 tsp olive oil
- 1 shallot, stripped and finely hacked
- 1 red (chime) pepper, deseeded and finely hacked
- 1 garlic clove, stripped and finely hacked
- 1 courgette (zucchini), stripped and finely hacked
- 1 tbsp. tomato purees (glue)
- ½ tsp gentle stew powder
- ¼ tsp ground cinnamon
- ¼ tsp ground cumin
- ½ tsp salt
- 1 × 400g (14oz) can hack tomatoes
- 1 x 400g (14oz) can chickpeas in water
- A little bunch of level leaf parsley (10g (1/3oz)), cleaved
- 4 medium eggs at room temperature

DIRECTIONS:

1. Heat the oil in a pan; include the shallot and red (ringer) pepper and fry delicately for 5 minutes. At that point include the garlic and courgette (zucchini) and cook for one more moment or two. Include the tomato puree (glue), flavors and salt and mix through.
2. Add the cleaved tomatoes and chickpeas (dousing alcohol and all) and increment the warmth to medium. With the top of the dish, stew the sauce for 30 minutes—ensure it is delicately rising all through and permit it to lessen in volume by around 33%.
3. Remove from the warmth and mix in the cleaved parsley.
4. Preheat the grill to 200°C/180°C fan/350°F.
5. When you are prepared to cook the eggs, bring the tomato sauce up to a delicate stew and move to a little broiler confirmation dish.
6. Crack the eggs on the dish and lower them delicately into the stew. Spread with thwart and prepare in the grill for 10-15 minutes. Serve the blend in unique dishes with the eggs coasting on the top.

NUTRITION:

- Calories 116 kcal
- Protein 6.97g
- Fat 5.22g
- Carbohydrates 13.14g

APPLE AND BLACKCURRANT PANCAKES

Preparation Time: 30 minutes
Cooking Time: 10 minutes
Servings: 4

INGREDIENTS:

- 2 apples cut into small chunks
- 2 cups of quick cooking oats
- 1 cup flour of your choice
- 1 tsp baking powder
- 2 tbsp. raw sugar, coconut sugar, or 2 tbsp. honey that is warm and easy to distribute
- 2 egg whites
- 1 ¼ cups of milk (or soy/rice/coconut)
- 2 tsp extra virgin olive oil
- A dash of salt
- For the berry topping:
- 1 cup blackcurrants, washed and stalks removed
- 3 tbsp. water (may use less)
- 2 tbsp. sugar (see above for types)

DIRECTIONS:

1. Place the ingredients for the topping in a small pot simmer, stirring frequently for about 10 minutes until it cooks down and the juices are released.

2. Take the dry ingredients and mix in a bowl. After, add the apples and the milk a bit at a time (you may not use it all), until it is a batter. Stiffly whisk the egg whites and then gently mix them into the pancake batter. Set aside in the refrigerator.

3. Pour one quarter of the oil onto a flat pan or flat griddle, and when hot, pour some of the batter into it in a pancake shape. When the pancakes start to have golden brown edges and form air bubbles, they may be ready to be gently flipped.

4. Test to be sure the bottom can lift away from the pan before actually flipping. Repeat for the next three pancakes. Top each pancake with the berries.

NUTRITION:

- Calories 337

FRUIT AND YOGHURT MUESLI

Preparation Time: 3 minutes
Cooking Time: 3 minutes
Servings: 1

INGREDIENTS:

- 100g plain Greek, coconut or soya yoghurt
- 100g of hulled and chopped strawberries
- 10g of cocoa nibs
- 15g chopped walnuts
- 40g of pitted and chopped Medjool dates
- 15g of coconut flakes or desiccated coconut
- 10g of buckwheat puffs
- 20g of buckwheat flakes

DIRECTIONS:

1. Mix together the cocoa nibs, buckwheat flakes, coconut flakes, buckwheat puffs, Medjool dates and walnuts. Add the yoghurt and strawberries when ready to serve.

NUTRITION:

- Kcal 368
- Net carbs 49g
- Fat 11.5g
- Fiber 7.4g
- Protein 16.54g

CHILAQUILES WITH GOCHUJANG

Preparation Time: 30 minutes
Cooking Time: 20 minutes
Servings: 2

INGREDIENTS:

- 1 dried ancho Chile
- 2 cups of water
- 1 cup squashed tomatoes
- 2 garlic cloves
- 1 teaspoon genuine salt
- 1/2 tablespoons gochujang
- 5 to 6 cups tortilla chips

- 3 big eggs
- 1 tablespoon olive oil
- Cotija cheese
- Cilantro, chopped
- Jalapeño
- Onion
- Avocado

DIRECTIONS:

1. Get the water to heat a pot. I cheated marginally and heated the water in an electric pot and emptied it into the pan. There's no sound unrivalled strategy here. Add the ancho Chile to the boiling water and drench for 15 minutes to give it an opportunity to stout up.

2. When completed, use tongs or a spoon to extricate Chile. Make sure to spare the water for the sauce! Nonetheless, on the off chance that you incidentally dump the water, it's not the apocalypse.

3. Mix the doused Chile, 1 cup of saved high temp water, squashed tomatoes, garlic, salt and gochujang until smooth.

4. Empty sauce into a large dish and warmth over medium warmth for 4 to 5 minutes. Lower the heat and include the tortilla chips. Mix the chips to cover with the sauce. In a different skillet, shower a teaspoon of oil and fry an egg on top, until the whites have settled. Plate the egg and cook the remainder of the eggs. If you are phenomenal at performing various tasks, you can likely sear the eggs while you heat the red sauce. I am not precisely so capable.

5. Top the chips with the seared eggs, cotija, hacked cilantro, jalapeños, onions and avocado. Serve right away.

NUTRITION:

- Calories 484kcal
- Protein 14.55g

- Fat 18.62g
- Carbohydrates 64.04g

TURMERIC PANCAKES WITH LEMON YOGURT SAUCE

Preparation Time: 45 minutes
Cooking Time: 15 minutes
Servings: 8 hotcakes

INGREDIENTS:
FOR THE YOGURT SAUCE

- 1 cup plain Greek yogurt
- 1garlic clove, minced
- 1 to 2 tablespoons lemon juice (from 1 lemon), to taste
- ¼ teaspoon ground turmeric
- 10 crisp mint leaves, minced
- 2 teaspoons lemon pizzazz (from 1 lemon)

FOR THE PANCAKES

- 2 teaspoons ground turmeric
- 1½ teaspoons ground cumin
- 1 teaspoon salt
- 1 teaspoon ground coriander
- ½ teaspoon garlic powder
- ½ teaspoon naturally ground dark pepper
- 1 head broccoli, cut into florets
- 3 big eggs, gently beaten
- 2 tablespoons plain unsweetened almond milk
- 1 cup almond flour
- 4 teaspoons coconut oil

DIRECTIONS:

1. Make the yogurt sauce. Mix the yogurt, garlic, lemon juice, turmeric, mint and pizzazz in a bowl. Taste and enjoy with more lemon juice, if possible. Keep in a safe spot or freeze until prepared to serve.
2. Make the pancakes. In a little bowl, mix the turmeric, cumin, salt, coriander, garlic and pepper.
3. Put the broccoli in a nourishment processor, and heartbeat until the florets are separated into little pieces. Move the broccoli to an big bowl and add the eggs, almond milk, and almond flour. Mix in the flavor blend and consolidate well.
4. Heat 1 teaspoon of the coconut oil in a non-stick dish over medium-low heat. Empty ¼ cup player into the skillet. Cook the hotcake until little air pockets start to show up superficially and the base is brilliant darker, 2 to 3 minutes. Flip over and cook the hotcake for 2 to 3 minutes more. To keep warm, move the cooked hotcakes to a stove safe dish and spot in a 200°F oven.
5. Keep making the staying 3 hotcakes, utilizing the rest of the oil and player.

NUTRITION:

- Calories 262
- Protein 11.68g
- Fat 19.28g
- Carbohydrates 12.06g

BUCKWHEAT PANCAKES WITH DARK CHOCOLATE SAUCE

Preparation Time: 5 minutes
Cooking Time: 20 minutes
Servings: 6-8

INGREDIENTS:

FOR THE PANCAKES YOU WILL NEED:

- 350ml milk
- 150g buckwheat flour
- 1 large egg
- 1 tbsp. extra virgin olive oil, for cooking

FOR THE CHOCOLATE SAUCE

- 100g dark chocolate (85 percent cocoa solids)
- 85ml milk
- 1 tbsp. double cream
- 1 tbsp. extra virgin olive oil
- To serve
- 400g strawberries, hulled and chopped
- 100g walnuts, chopped

DIRECTIONS:

1. To make the pancake batter, place all of the ingredients apart from the olive oil in a blender. Blend until you have a smooth batter. It should not be too thick or too runny. (You can store any excess batter in an airtight container for up to 5 days in your fridge. Be sure to mix well before using again.)

2. To make the chocolate sauce, melt the chocolate in a heatproof bowl over a pan of simmering water. Once melted, mix in the milk, whisking thoroughly and then add the double cream and olive oil. You can keep the sauce warm by leaving the water in the pan simmering on a very low heat until your pancakes are ready.

3. To make the pancakes heat a heavy-bottomed frying pan until it starts to smoke, then add the olive oil.

4. Pour some of the batter into the center of the pan, then tip the excess batter around it until you have covered the whole surface, you may have to add a little more batter to achieve this. You will only need to cook the pancake for 1 minute or so on each side if your pan is hot enough.

5. Once you can see it going brown around the edges, use a spatula to loosen the pancake around its edge, and then flip it over. Try to flip in one action to avoid breaking it.

6. Cook for one minute or so on the other side. Transfer to a plate.

7. Place some strawberries in the center, then roll up the pancake. Continue until you have made as many pancakes as you need.

8. Spoon over a generous amount of sauce and sprinkle over some chopped walnuts.

9. You may find that your first efforts are too fat or fall apart but once you find the consistency of your batter that works best for you and you get your technique perfected, you'll be making them like a professional. Practice makes perfect in this case.

NUTRITION:

- Calories 109
- Total Fat 6g
- Cholesterol 16mg
- Sodium 139mg

- Carbohydrates 12g
- Fiber 2g
- Sugar 3g
- Protein 3g

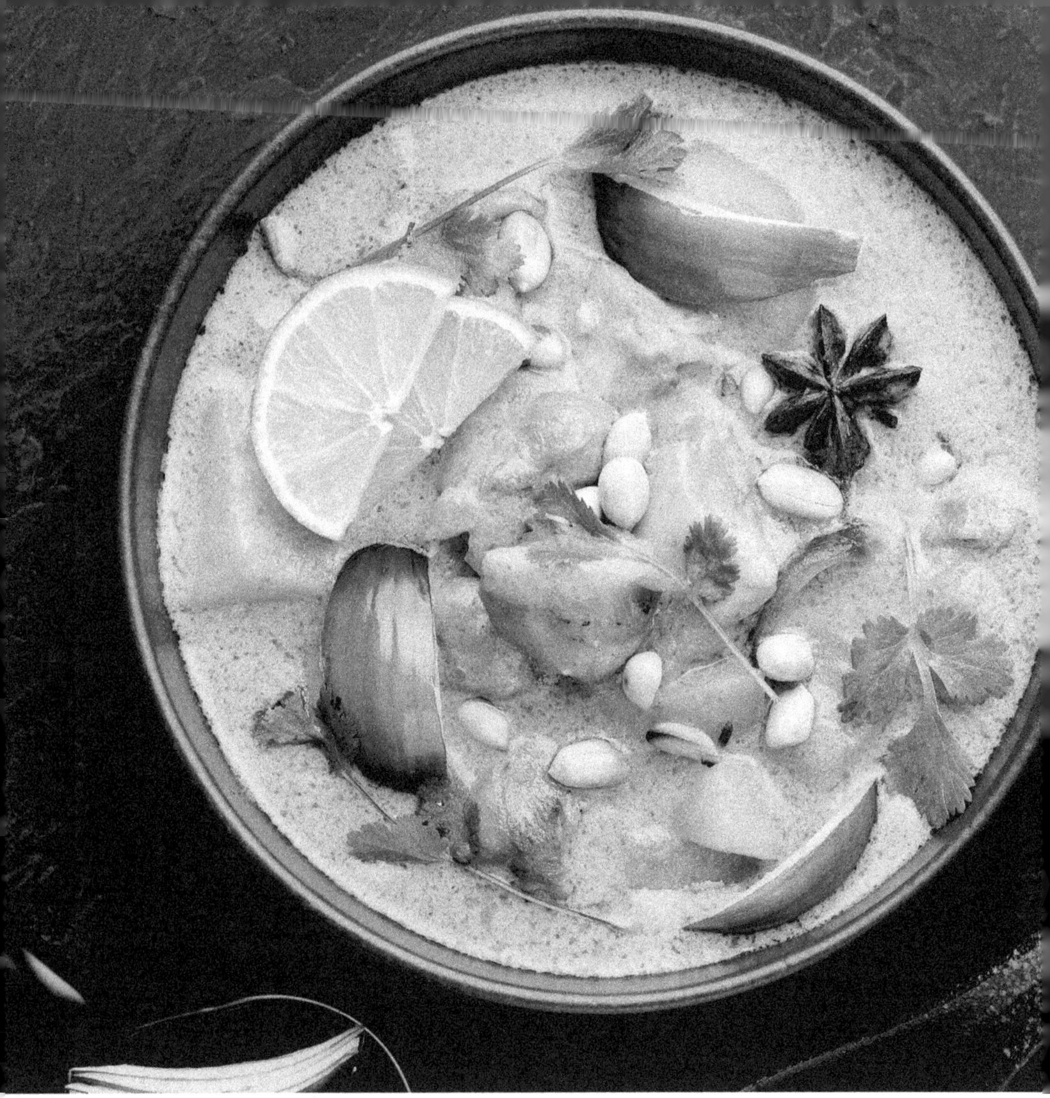

CHAPTER
04

LUNCH RECIPES

Chapter 4: Lunch Recipes

FRAGRANT ASIAN HOTPOT

Preparation Time: 30 minutes
Cooking Time: 10 minutes
Servings: 2

INGREDIENTS:

- 1 teaspoon tomato puree
- 1-star anise, crushed (or 1/4 teaspoon anise)
- A small handful (10g) of parsley, finely chopped stalks
- A small handful of coriander (10g), finely chopped stalks
- Juice from 1/2 lime
- 500 ml chicken broth, fresh or made from 1 cube
- 1/2 carrot, peeled and cut into matches
- 50g broccoli, cut into small roses
- 50g bean sprouts
- 100g raw tiger prawns
- 100g hard tofu, chopped
- 50g rice noodles, cooked according to the instructions on the packaging
- 50g of boiled water chestnuts, drained
- 20g chopped ginger sushi
- 1 tablespoon of good quality miso paste

DIRECTIONS:

1. Place in a large saucepan the tomato purée, star anise, parsley stalks, coriander stalks, lime juice and chicken stock and bring 10 minutes to a simmer.

2. Stir in the cabbage, broccoli, prawns, tofu, noodles, and water chestnuts and cook gently until the prawns are finished. Remove from heat and whisk in the ginger sushi and the paste miso.

3. Serve sprinkled with the leaves of the parsley and coriander.

NUTRITION:

- Calories 253Cal
- Fat 7.35g
- Carbohydrates 29.99g
- Protein 19.39
- Fiber 6g

Prawn Pasta

Preparation Time: 1 hour
Cooking Time: 45 minutes
Servings: 6-7

INGREDIENTS:

- 125-150g Raw or cooked prawns (Ideally ruler prawns)
- 65g Buckwheat pasta
- 1 tbsp Extra virgin olive oil
- For arrabbiata sauce
- 40g Red onion, finely slashed
- 1garlic clove, finely slashed
- 30g Celery, finely slashed
- 1 Bird's eye bean stew, finely hacked
- 1 tsp Dried blended herbs
- 1 tsp Extra virgin olive oil
- 2 tbsp White wine (discretionary)
- 400g Tinned slashed tomatoes
- 1 tbsp Chopped parsley

DIRECTIONS:

1. Fry the onion, garlic, celery and bean stew and dried herbs in the oil over a medium-low warmth for 1-2 minutes. Turn the heat up to medium, include the wine and cook for one moment. Include the tomatoes and leave the sauce to stew over a medium-low warmth for 20-30 minutes, until it has a pleasant creamy consistency. On the off chance that you feel the sauce is getting too thick just include a little water.

2. While the sauce is cooking, carry a container of water to the bubble and cook the pasta as per the bundle guidelines. At the point when prepared just as you would prefer, channel, hurl with the olive oil and keep in the container until required.

3. On the off that you are utilizing crude prawns mix them to the sauce and bake for a further 3-4 minutes until it has turned pink and dark, including the parsley and serve. If you are utilizing cooked prawns, include them with the parsley, carry the sauce to the bubble and help.

4. Add pasta to the sauce, blend altogether yet tenderly and serve.

NUTRITION:

- Calories 335Cal
- Fat 12g
- Carbs 38g
- Sugar 0g
- Protein 19g
- Fiber 0g

BAKED SALMON WITH SPICY CELERY

Preparation Time: 5 minutes
Cooking Time: 15 minutes
Servings: 1

INGREDIENTS:

- 125-150g Skinned Salmon
- 1 tsp extra virgin olive oil
- 1 tsp ground turmeric
- 1/4 Juice of a lemon
- For the fiery celery
- 1 tsp extra virgin olive oil
- 40g Red onion, finely slashed
- 60g Tinned green lentils
- 1garlic clove, finely slashed
- 1 cm fresh ginger, finely slashed
- 1 Bier's eye bean stew, finely slashed
- 150g Celery cut into 2cm lengths
- 1 tsp Mild curry powder
- 130g Tomato, cut into eight wedges
- 100 ml Chicken or vegetable stock
- 1 tbsp. Chopped parsley

DIRECTIONS:

1. Heat the grill to 200°C/gas mark 6.
2. Start with the fiery celery. Warmth a skillet over medium-low heat, include the olive oil, at that point the onion, garlic, ginger, bean stew and celery. Fry tenderly for 2-3 minutes or until mollified however not hued, at that point include the curry powder and cook for a further moment.
3. Add the red tomato then the stock and lentils and stew delicately for 10 minutes. You might need to increment or decrease the cooking time contingent upon how crunchy you like your celery.
4. Meanwhile, blend the turmeric, oil and lemon squeeze and rub over the salmon.
5. Place on a heating plate and cook for 8–10 minutes.
6. To complete, mix the parsley through the celery and present with the salmon.

NUTRITION:

- Calories 25
- Immersed fat 1.3g
- Cholesterol 28mg
- Sodium 20mg
- Potassium 93mg
- Starches 2g
- Folate 79mcg
- Calcium 19mg

THE BELL PEPPER FIESTA

Preparation Time: 10 minutes
Cooking Time: 0 minutes
Servings: 4

INGREDIENTS:

- 2 tablespoons dill, chopped
- 1 yellow onion, chopped
- 1 pound multi colored peppers, cut, halved, seeded and cut into thin strips
- 3 tablespoons organic olive oil
- 2 ½ tablespoons white wine vinegar
- Black pepper to taste

DIRECTIONS:

1. Take a bowl and mix in sweet pepper, onion, dill, pepper, oil, vinegar and toss well.
2. Divide between bowls and serve.
3. Enjoy!

NUTRITION:

- Calories 120
- Fat 3g
- Carbohydrates 1g
- Protein 6g

DAL WITH KALE, RED ONIONS AND BUCKWHEAT

Preparation Time: 5 minutes
Cooking Time: 20 minutes
Servings: 2

INGREDIENTS:

- 1 teaspoon of extra virgin olive oil
- 1 teaspoon of mustard seeds
- 40g red onions, finely chopped
- 1 garlic clove, very finely chopped
- 1 teaspoon very finely chopped ginger
- 1 Thai chili, very finely chopped
- 1 teaspoon curry mixture
- 2 teaspoons turmeric
- 300ml vegetable broth
- 40g red lentils
- 50g kale, chopped
- 50ml coconut milk
- 50g buckwheat

DIRECTIONS:

1. Heat oil in a pan
2. Add the curry powder and 1 teaspoon of turmeric, mix well.
3. Add the vegetable stock, bring to the boil.
4. Add the lentils and cook them for 25 to 30 minutes until they are ready.
5. Then add the kale and coconut milk and simmer for 5 minutes. The Dal is ready.

NUTRITION:

- Calories 289Cal
- Fat 18g
- Carbs 28g
- Protein 13g
- Fiber 10g

SPICED UP PUMPKIN SEEDS BOWLS

Preparation Time: 10 minutes
Cooking Time: 20 minutes
Servings: 4

INGREDIENTS:

- ½ tablespoon chili powder
- ½ teaspoon cayenne
- 2 cups pumpkin seeds
- 2 teaspoons lime juice

DIRECTIONS:

1. Spread pumpkin seeds over lined baking sheet; add lime juice, cayenne and chili powder.
2. Toss well.
3. Pre-heat your oven to 275 degrees F.
4. Roast in your oven for 20 minutes and transfer to small bowls.
5. Serve and enjoy!

NUTRITION:

- Calories 170
- Fat 3g
- Carbohydrates 10g
- Protein 6g

CHICKEN & BEAN CASSEROLE

Preparation Time: 5 minutes
Cooking Time: 40 minutes
Servings: 2

INGREDIENTS:

- 400g (14oz) chopped tomatoes
- 400g (14 oz) tinned cannellini beans or haricot beans
- 8 chicken thighs, skin removed
- 2 carrots, peeled and finely chopped
- 2 red onions, chopped
- 4 sticks of celery
- 4 large mushrooms
- 2 red peppers bell peppers, deseeded and chopped
- 1 garlic clove
- 2 tablespoons soy sauce
- 1 tablespoon olive oil
- 1.75 liters (3 pints) chicken stock broth
- 509 calories per serving

DIRECTIONS:

1. Heat the olive oil. Add the garlic and onions and cook for 5 minutes. Add in the chicken, carrots, cannellini beans, celery, red peppers bell peppers and mushrooms. Pour in the stock broth soy sauce and tomatoes. Bring it to the boil. Serve.

NUTRITION:

- Calories 330Cal
- Fat 25g
- Carbs 32g
- Protein 16g
- Fiber 20g

SERRANO HAM & ROCKET ARUGULA

Preparation Time: 5 minutes
Cooking Time: 60 minutes
Servings: 2

INGREDIENTS:

- 175g (6oz) Serrano ham
- 125g (4oz) rocket arugula leaves
- 2 tablespoons olive oil
- 1 tablespoon orange juice

DIRECTIONS:

1. Pour the oil and juice into a bowl and toss the rocket arugula in the mixture. Serve the rocket onto plates and top it off with the ham.

NUTRITION:

- Calories 165.3
- Protein 7.0g
- Carbs 9.9g
- Fat 11.2g

COUNTRY CHICKEN BREASTS

Preparation Time: 10 minutes
Cooking Time: 45 minutes
Servings: 2

INGREDIENTS:

- 2 medium green apples, diced
- 1 small red onion, finely diced
- 1 small green bell pepper, chopped
- 3 garlic cloves, minced
- 2 tablespoons dried currants
- 1 tablespoon curry powder
- 1 teaspoon turmeric
- 1 teaspoon ground ginger
- ¼ teaspoon chili pepper flakes
- 1 can (14 ½ ounce) diced tomatoes
- 6 skinless, boneless chicken breasts, halved
- ½ cup chicken broth
- 1 cup long-grain white rice
- 1-pound large raw shrimp, shelled and deveined
- Salt and pepper to taste
- Chopped parsley
- 1/3 cup slivered almonds

DIRECTIONS:

1. Rinse chicken, pat dry and set aside.
2. In a large crockpot, combine apples, onion, bell pepper, garlic, currants, curry powder, turmeric, ginger, and chili pepper flakes. Stir in tomatoes.
3. Arrange chicken, overlapping pieces slightly, on top of tomato mixture.
4. Pour in broth and do not mix or stir.
5. Cover and cook for 6-7 hours on low.
6. Preheat oven to 200 degrees F.
7. Carefully transfer chicken to an oven-safe plate, cover lightly, and keep warm in the oven.
8. Stir rice into remaining liquid. Increase cooker heat setting to high; cover and cook, stirring once or twice, until rice is almost tender to bite, 30 to 35 minutes. Stir in shrimp, cover and cook until shrimp are opaque in center, about 10 more minutes.

9. Meanwhile, toast almonds in a small pan over medium heat until golden brown, 5-8 minutes, stirring occasionally. Set aside.

10. Mound in a warm serving dish and arrange chicken on top. Sprinkle with parsley and almonds.

NUTRITION:

- Calories 155
- Carbs 13.9g
- Protein 17.4g
- Fat 3.8g

APPLES AND CABBAGE MIX

Preparation Time: 5 minutes
Cooking Time: 0 minutes
Servings: 4

INGREDIENTS:

- 2 cored and cubed green apples
- 2tbsps. Balsamic vinegar
- ½ tsp. caraway seeds
- 2tbsps. olive oil
- Black pepper
- 1 shredded red cabbage head

DIRECTIONS:

1. In a bowl, combine the cabbage with the apples and the other ingredients, toss and serve.

NUTRITION:

- Calories 165
- Fat 7.4g
- Carbs 26g
- Protein 2.6g
- Sugars 2.6g
- Sodium 19mg

Thyme Mushrooms

Preparation Time: 10 minutes
Cooking Time: 45 minutes
Servings: 2

INGREDIENTS:

- 1 tbsp. chopped thyme
- 2tbsps. olive oil
- 2tbsps. chopped parsley
- 4 minced garlic cloves
- Black pepper
- 2 lbs. halved white mushrooms

DIRECTIONS:

1. In a baking pan, combine the mushrooms with the garlic and the other ingredients, toss, introduce in the oven and cook at 400°F for 30 minutes.

2. Divide between plates and serve.

NUTRITION:

- Calories 251
- Fat 9.3g
- Carbs 13.2g
- Protein 6g
- Sugars 0.8g
- Sodium 37mg

CINNAMON BUCKWHEAT BOWLS

Preparation Time: 5 minutes
Cooking Time: 15 minutes
Servings: 1

INGREDIENTS:

- ½ cup buckwheat groats, rinsed
- ½ cup almond milk or milk of choice
- ½ teaspoon cinnamon
- ½ cup water
- ½ teaspoon vanilla
- Honey to serve
- Sliced fruit to serve

DIRECTIONS:

1. In a small saucepan, add washed buckwheat grains, water, almond milk, cinnamon, and vanilla. Boil and then simmer and cover with a lid. Cook over low heat for 10 minutes.

2. Turn off the heat and steam, covered, for an additional 5 minutes.

3. Pour with a fork and divide into a bowl. Fill with fruit slices, sprinkle more milk and chopped honey if desired.

NUTRITION:

- Calories 182
- Fat 1g
- Carbohydrates 34g
- Protein 6.7g

SIRTFOOD SALMON SALAD

Preparation Time: 10 minutes
Cooking Time: 0 minutes
Servings: 1

INGREDIENTS:

- 1 cup rocket
- 2 oz. chicory leaves
- 1 tablespoon capers
- 3 oz. avocado, peeled, stoned and sliced
- 3.5 oz. smoked salmon slices
- 1/8 cup walnuts, chopped
- 1 large Medjool date, pitted and chopped
- Juice of ¼ lemon
- 1 tablespoon extra-virgin olive oil
- 3/8 cup parsley, chopped
- ½ oz. celery leaves
- ¼ cup red onion, sliced

DIRECTIONS:

1. Place the salad leaves in a big bowl. Mix all the other ingredients and serve on the leaves.

NUTRITION:

- Calories 194
- Fat 9g
- Carbohydrates 4.5g
- Protein 21g

ARUGULA, EGG, AND CHARRED ASPARAGUS SALAD

Preparation Time: 5 minutes
Cooking Time: 15 minutes
Servings: 4

INGREDIENTS:

- 12 oz. medium asparagus, trimmed
- ½ teaspoon black pepper, divided
- 4 large eggs in shells
- 1 tablespoon fresh lemon juice
- 5 oz. baby arugula
- 1 tablespoon extra-virgin olive oil
- 1 tablespoon water
- ¼ cup plain whole-milk Greek yogurt
- 1 teaspoon kosher salt, divided

DIRECTIONS:

1. Preheat broiler to high.
2. Bring a small saucepan filled with water to a boil. Carefully add eggs. Cook 8 minutes. Place eggs in a bowl filled with ice water and let stand for 2 minutes. Peel eggs, cut into quarters, and sprinkle with ¼ teaspoon salt and 1/8 teaspoon pepper.
3. Combine olive oil, ¼ teaspoon salt, ¼ teaspoon pepper, and asparagus on a baking sheet. Spread in a single layer in pan. Broil 3 minutes or until lightly charred. Remove asparagus mixture from pan and cut into 2 inch pieces.
4. Combine remaining ¼ teaspoon salt, remaining 1/8 teaspoon pepper, yogurt, juice, and 1 tablespoon water in a medium bowl, stirring with a whisk. Add arugula and toss. Arrange arugula mixture on a platter. Top with asparagus mixture and eggs. Enjoy!

NUTRITION:

- Calories 147
- Fat 9.1g
- Carbohydrates 6g
- Protein 10g

Spring Vegetable and Quinoa Salad with Bacon

Preparation Time: 5 minutes
Cooking Time: 10 minutes
Servings: 4

INGREDIENTS:

- 1 ¾ cups ginger-coconut quinoa
- 2.5 cups fresh asparagus, cut diagonally into 1 inch pieces
- 3 center-cut bacon slices, chopped
- 1 tablespoon unsalted butter
- 3 tablespoons cider vinegar
- ½ cup frozen green peas
- 2 teaspoons whole-grain Dijon mustard
- 5 oz. baby spinach
- 3 tablespoons sliced almonds, toasted
- 1 teaspoon black pepper
- 1 tablespoon fresh thyme leaves
- 1 tablespoon chopped fresh tarragon
- ½ cup chopped fresh flat-leaf parsley

DIRECTIONS:

1. Boil a large pot filled with water. Add asparagus and peas. Boil 2 minutes, then drain. Plunge into a bowl of ice water. Drain.

2. Cook the bacon in a large saucepan over medium-high heat, stirring occasionally. Remove bacon from pan with a slotted spoon. Set aside. Add vinegar, butter, and Dijon mustard to drippings in pan, stirring with a whisk until butter melts. Add quinoa and pepper to pan. Cook 1 minute. Place quinoa mixture in a medium bowl. Add asparagus mixture, parsley, tarragon, thyme, and spinach, tossing to combine. Divide quinoa mixture among 4 plates; sprinkle evenly with reserved bacon and almonds.

NUTRITION:

- Calories 263
- Fat 9.8g
- Carbohydrates 28g
- Protein 7g

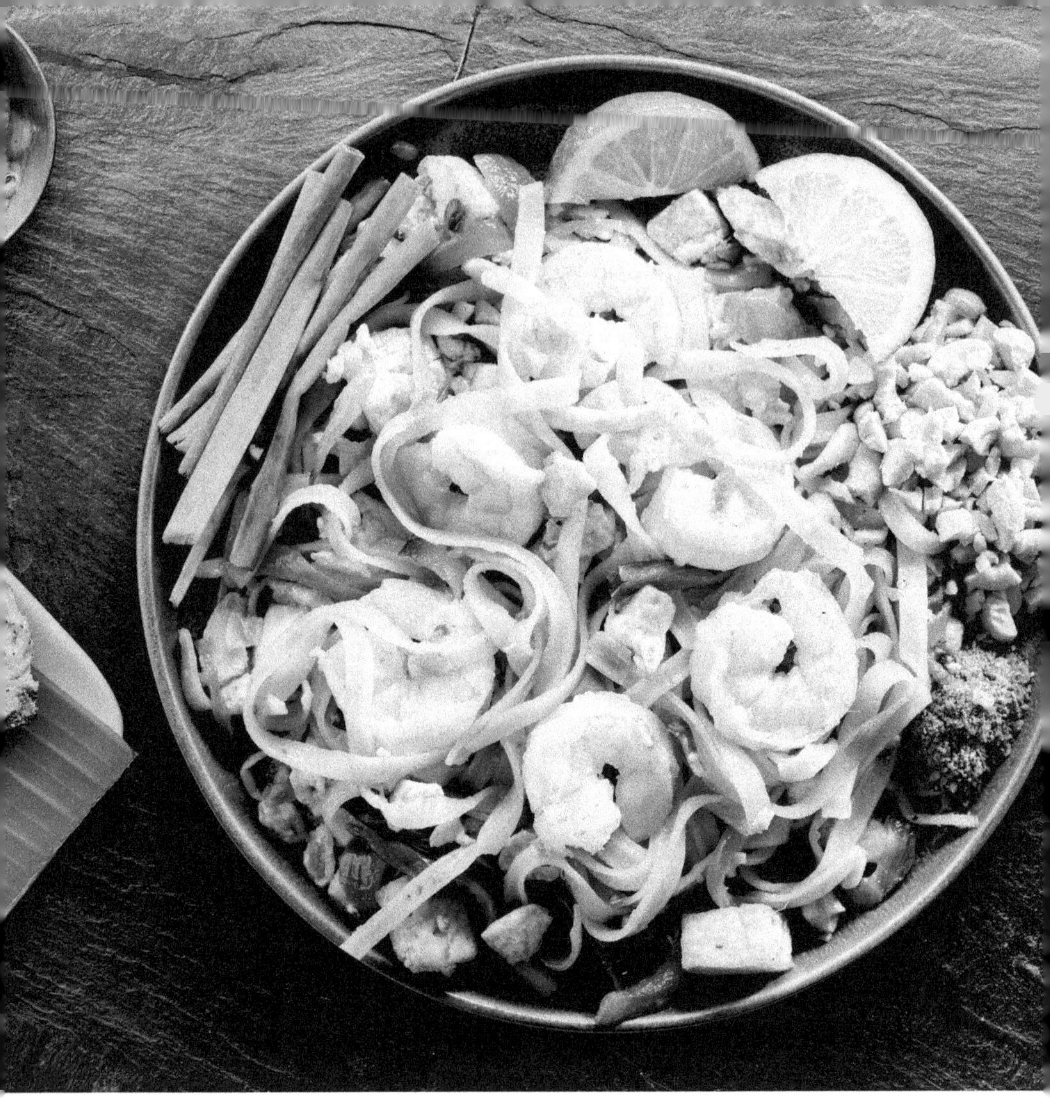

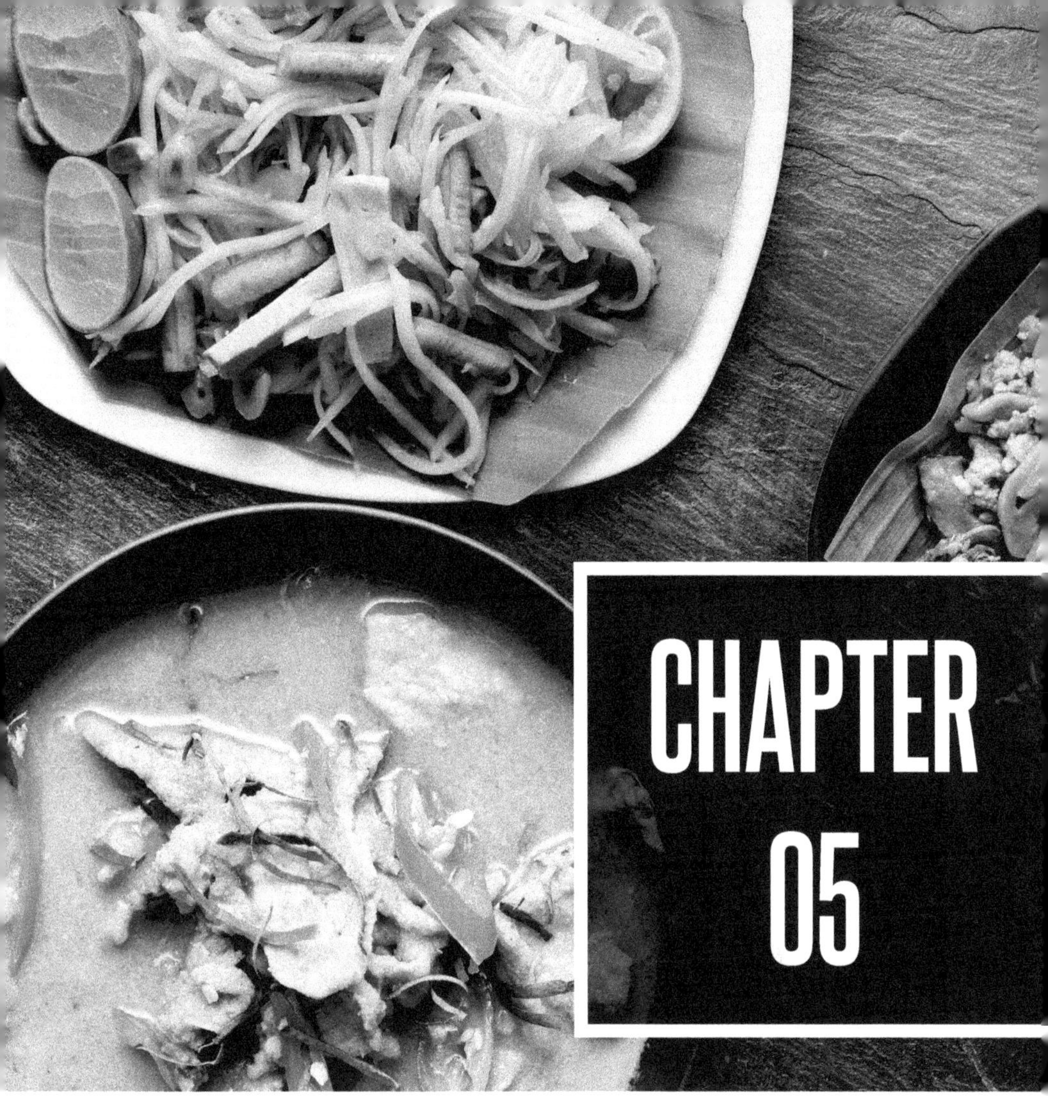

CHAPTER 05

DINNER RECIPES

Chapter5: Dinner Recipes

CHICKEN WITH RED ONION AND BLACK CABBAGE

Preparation Time: 10 minutes
Cooking Time: 15 minutes
Servings: 2-4

INGREDIENTS:

- 120g of chicken breast
- 130g of tomatoes
- 1 chilli pepper
- 1 tablespoon of capers
- 5g of parsley
- Lemon juice
- 2 tbsp. Extra virgin olive oil
- 2 teaspoons of turmeric
- 50g of cabbage
- 20g of red onion
- 1 teaspoon fresh ginger
- 50g of buckwheat

DIRECTIONS:

1. Marinate the chicken breast for 10 minutes with 1/4 of lemon juice, 1 tablespoon of extra virgin olive oil and 1 teaspoon of turmeric powder.
2. Cut 130g of chopped tomatoes, remove the inside, season with Bird's Eye pepper, 1 tablespoon of capers, 1 teaspoon of turmeric and 1 of extra virgin olive oil, 1/4 of lemon juice and 5g of parsley chopped.
3. Fry the chicken breast, dripped from the marinade, on a high flame for one minute on each side, then put it in the oven for about 10 minutes at 220°C.
4. Let it rest covered with aluminum foil.
5. Steam the chopped kale for 5 minutes.
6. Sauté a red onion, a teaspoon of grated fresh ginger and a teaspoon of extra virgin olive oil; add the cooked cabbage and cook for a minute on the fire.
7. Boil the buckwheat with a teaspoon of turmeric, drain and serve with chicken, tomatoes and chopped cabbage.

NUTRITION:

- Calories 52
- Carbs 12g
- Fat 0g
- Protein 2g

TURKEY WITH CAULIFLOWER COUSCOUS

Preparation Time: 15 minutes
Cooking Time: 0 minutes
Servings: 2-4

INGREDIENTS:

- 150g of turkey
- 150g of cauliflower
- 40g of red onion
- 1 teaspoon fresh ginger
- 1 bird's eye pepper
- 1 garlic clove
- 3 tablespoons of extra virgin olive oil
- 2 teaspoons of turmeric
- 30g of dried tomatoes
- 10g of parsley
- Dried sage to taste
- 1 tablespoon of capers
- 1/4 of fresh lemon juice

DIRECTIONS:

1. Blend the raw cauliflower tops and cook them in a teaspoon of extra virgin olive oil, garlic, red onion, chilli pepper, ginger and a teaspoon of turmeric.

2. Leave to flavor for a minute, then add the chopped sun-dried tomatoes and 5g of parsley over the heat.

3. Season the turkey slice with a teaspoon of extra virgin olive oil, the dried sage and cook it in another teaspoon of extra virgin olive oil.

4. Once ready, season with a tablespoon of capers, 1/4 of lemon juice, 5g of parsley, a tablespoon of water and add the cauliflower.

NUTRITION:

- Calories 394
- Carbs 28g
- Fat 20g
- Protein 28g

FARRO WITH VEGETABLES AND CHICKEN

Preparation Time: 25 minutes
Cooking Time: 30 minutes
Servings: 2-4

INGREDIENTS:

- 320g of spelled
- 2 courgettes
- 3 carrots
- 2 potatoes
- 150g of green beans
- 150g of peas
- 300g of chicken
- 1 onion
- 2 garlic cloves
- Extra virgin olive oil
- Parsley
- Salt to taste

DIRECTIONS:

1. Wash the spelled and cook it in boiling salted water for 25 minutes.

2. Wash and cut the vegetables.

3. In a pan, brown the onion and the garlic cloves minced in 3 tablespoons of oil, add the diced chicken, brown it, sprinkle with a little white wine, let it evaporate, add 1 ladle of broth, salt to taste and cook for 20 minutes.

4. At this point add the vegetables and continue cooking for 10 minutes.

5. Drain the spelled and add it to the chicken and vegetables. Mix and cook for a few minutes over low heat, add chopped parsley and serve.

NUTRITION:

- Calories 145
- Carbs 19g
- Fat 6g
- Protein 4g

Eggplant Salsa

Preparation Time: 10 minutes
Cooking Time: 10 minutes
Servings: 4

INGREDIENTS:

- 1 and ½ cups tomatoes, chopped
- 3 cups eggplant, cubed
- A drizzle of olive oil
- 2 teaspoons capers
- 6 ounces' green olives, pitted and sliced
- 4garlic cloves, minced
- 2 teaspoons balsamic vinegar
- 1 tablespoon basil, chopped
- Black pepper to the taste

DIRECTIONS:

1. Heat a saucepan with the oil medium-high heat, add eggplant, stir and cook for 5 minutes.

2. Add tomatoes, capers, olives, garlic, vinegar, basil and black pepper, toss, cook for 5 minutes more, divide into small cups and serve cold.

NUTRITION:

- Calories 120
- Fat 6
- Fiber 5
- Carbs 9
- Protein 7

Yummy Peanut Chicken

Preparation Time: 10 minutes.
Cooking Time: 20 minutes
Servings: 4

INGREDIENTS:

- 16 ounces chicken breast
- 2 red bell peppers, diced
- 2 green onions, diced
- 1 tablespoon ginger, grated
- ½ teaspoon cayenne pepper
- ½ cup crunchy organic peanut butter
- ¼ cup coconut aminos
- Coconut oil

DIRECTIONS:

1. Cut chicken breast into 1" cubes and sprinkle with salt.
2. Heat 2 tablespoons coconut oil in skillet over medium heat.
3. Brown chicken breast, remove to plate.
4. In same skillet add bell peppers, green onions, and ginger and sauté for 4 minutes.
5. Return chicken to pan, mix, add peanut butter, coconut aminos and cayenne pepper.
6. Stir-fry ingredients for 3 minutes and cover, reduce heat to low and cook for 10 minutes.

NUTRITION:

- Calories 439
- Fat 24
- Sodium 152 (mg)
- Carbs 11
- Sugar 4
- Protein 43

Italian White Beans

Preparation Time: 10 minutes
Cooking Time: 20 minutes
Servings: 4

INGREDIENTS:

- 2 cups white beans, drained
- 1 onion, minced
- 4 garlic cloves, minced
- 2 cups organic tomato sauce
- 1 teaspoon oregano
- 1 teaspoon black pepper
- 1 teaspoon salt
- Coconut oil

DIRECTIONS:

1. Heat 2 tablespoons coconut oil in a skillet.
2. Add garlic and onion and sauté for 2 minutes.
3. Add white beans, sauté for 5 minutes.
4. Add tomato sauce, salt, cover and cook for 10 minutes.
5. Add oregano and black pepper, remove from heat.

NUTRITION:

- Calories 444
- Fat 8
- Sodium 1241 (mg)
- Carbs 72
- Sugar 9
- Protein 26

CASSEROLE WITH SPINACH AND EGGPLANT

Preparation Time: 10 minutes
Cooking Time: 45 minutes
Servings: 6

INGREDIENTS:

- 1-piece Eggplant
- 2 pieces Onion
- 3 tablespoons Olive oil
- 450g Spinach (fresh)
- 4 pieces Tomatoes
- 2 pieces Egg
- 60 ml Almond milk
- 2 teaspoons Lemon juice
- 4 tablespoon Almond flour

DIRECTIONS:

1. Preheat the oven to 200°C.
2. Cut the eggplants, onions and tomatoes into slices and sprinkle salt on the eggplant slices.
3. Brush the eggplants and onions with olive oil and fry them in a grill pan.
4. Shrink the spinach in a large saucepan over moderate heat and drain in a sieve.
5. Put the vegetables in layers in a greased baking dish: first the eggplant, then the spinach and then the onion and the tomato. Repeat this again.
6. Whisk eggs with almond milk, lemon juice, salt and pepper and pour over the vegetables.
7. Sprinkle almond flour over the dish and bake in the oven for about 30 to 40 minutes.

NUTRITION:

- Calories 139.9
- Cholesterol 72
- Carbohydrate 21.5g
- Protein 10.3g

Courgette And Broccoli Soup

Preparation Time: 15 minutes
Cooking Time: 15 minutes
Servings: 6

INGREDIENTS:

- 2 tablespoon Coconut oil
- 1-piece Red onion
- 2 garlic cloves
- 300g Broccoli
- 1-piece Zucchini
- 750 ml vegetable broth

DIRECTIONS:

1. Finely chop the onion and garlic, cut the broccoli into florets and the zucchini into slices.
2. Melt the coconut oil in a soup pot and fry the onion with the garlic.
3. Cook the zucchini for a few minutes.
4. Add broccoli and vegetable broth and simmer for about 5 minutes.
5. Puree the soup with a hand blender and season with salt and pepper.

NUTRITION:

- Calories 115
- Carbohydrates 17g
- Protein 5g

SUPER-SPEEDY PRAWN RISOTTO

Preparation Time: 10 minutes
Cooking Time: 25 minutes
Servings: 4

INGREDIENTS:

- 100g Diced Onion
- 2 X 250g packs whole-grain Rice & Quinoa
- 200g Frozen Garden Peas
- 2 x 150g packs Cooked and Peeled King Prawns
- 1/285g Tote water-cress

DIRECTIONS:

1. Heating 1 tablespoon coconut oil in a skillet on medium-high heat and then put in 100g Diced Onion; cook 5 minutes. Insert 2 x 250g packs whole-grain Rice & Quinoa along with 175ml hot vegetable stock (or plain water); together side 200g suspended Garden Peas. Gently split using rice using a wooden spoon. Cover and cook 3 minutes, stirring occasionally, you can add 2 x 150g packs Cooked and Peeled King Prawns. Cook for 12 minutes before prawns, peas, and rice have been piping hot, and the majority of the liquid was consumed. Remove from heat. Chop 1/2 x 85g tote water-cress and stir throughout; up to taste. Top with watercress leaves and pepper to function.

NUTRITION:

- Calories 456
- Protein 5
- Carbohydrate 23
- Fat 6

MISO MARINATED COD WITH STIR-FRIED GREENS AND SESAME

Preparation Time: 25 minutes
Cooking Time: 35 minutes
Servings: 1

INGREDIENTS:

- 1 x 7-ounce Skinless cod fillet
- 1 tablespoon Mirin
- 3 ½ teaspoon Miso
- ¾ cup Kale (roughly chopped)
- 1 tablespoon Extra virgin olive oil
- 1/8 cup Red onion (sliced)
- 3/8 cup Celery (sliced)
- ¼ cup Buckwheat
- 1 Bird's eye chili (finely chopped)
- 1 Garlic clove (finely chopped)
- 1 teaspoon Finely chopped fresh ginger
- 1 teaspoon Sesame seeds
- 3/8 cup Green beans
- 2 tablespoons Parsley (roughly chopped)
- 1 tablespoon Tamari
- 1 teaspoon Ground turmeric

DIRECTIONS:

1. Add 1 teaspoon of oil, the mirin and miso into a bowl and mix together. Rub the mixture all over the cod and leave it for 30 minutes to marinate. Heat your oven to 220°C or 425°F. Bake the cod for approx. ten minutes.

2. Add the remaining oil into a large frypan or wok over medium heat. Once hot, add the onions and stir-fry for 3 minutes, then add the garlic, celery, green beans, ginger, chili, and kale. Stir and fry until the kale is well cooked and tender. Add a little water to the pan if needed to aid the cooking process.

3. Cook the buckwheat following the instruction on the packet, add the turmeric three minutes to the end.

4. Add the sesame seeds, tamari, and parsley to the stir fry. Serve with the fish and the greens.

NUTRITION:

- Calories 213
- Fat 4
- Protein 9

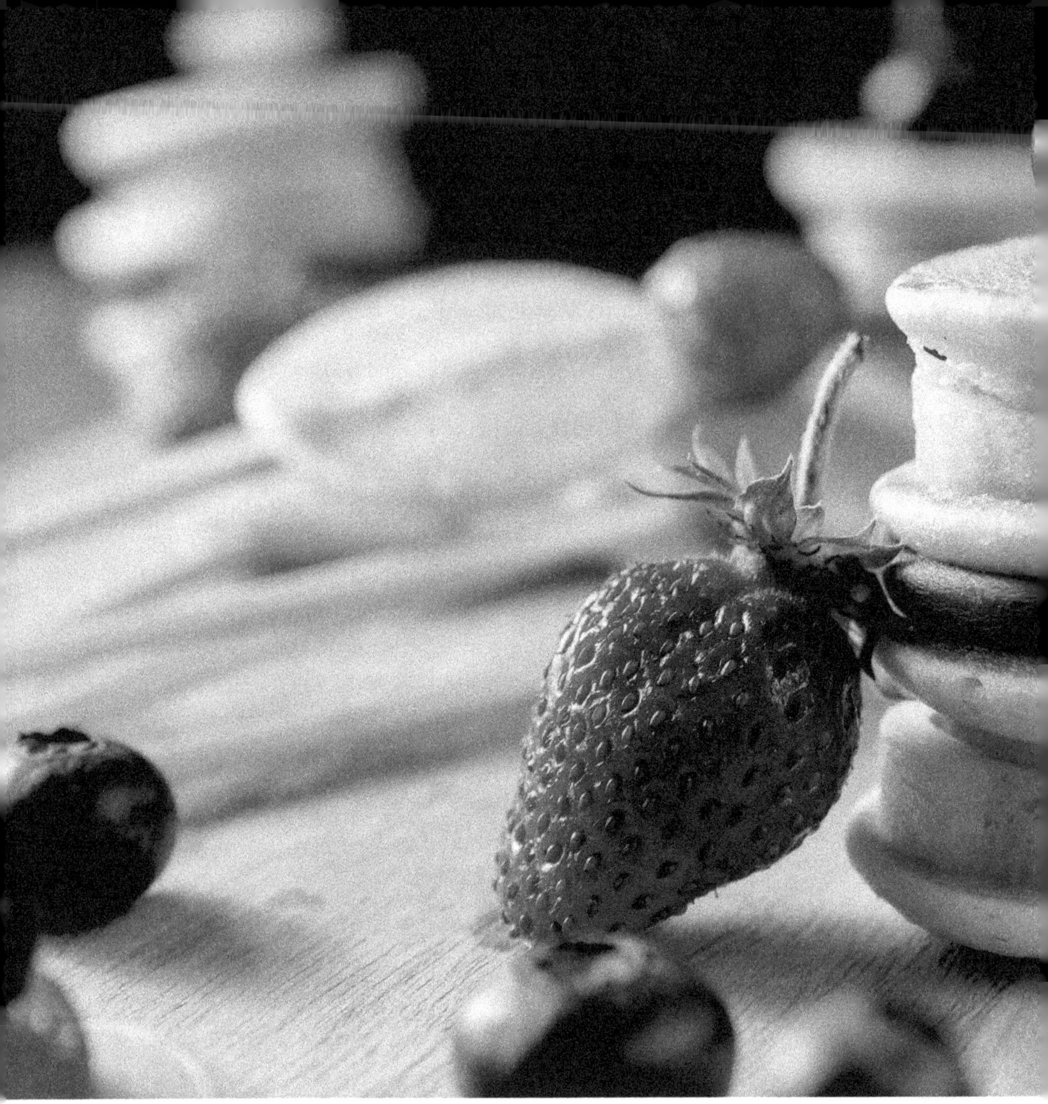

CHAPTER 06

SNACK AND DESSERT

Chapter 6: Snacks and Dessert

Pancake Skewers with Fruits

Preparation Time: 0 minutes
Cooking Time: 30 minutes
Servings: 4

Ingredients:

- 100g dark chocolate (at least 70% cocoa)
- 3 bananas
- 200g buttermilk
- 100g yogurt (3.5% fat)
- 3 eggs
- 3 tbsp. rapeseed oil
- 100g 5-grain flakes (or oat flakes)
- 100g wholemeal spelled flour
- ½ tsp. baking soda
- 1 tsp. baking powder
- 1 tbsp. whole cane sugar
- 150g strawberries
- 2 handfuls blueberries

Directions:

1. Chop the chocolate and melt over a warm water bath. Peel bananas, slice them, pull them through the chocolate and let them dry on baking paper.

2. Mix the buttermilk, yogurt, eggs, and 1 tablespoon of rapeseed oil. Chop the 5-grain flakes very finely in a blender, then add the flour, baking soda, baking powder, and sugar to another bowl and mix. Add liquid ingredients and make a smooth dough. Let it rest for about 10 minutes.

3. In the meantime, clean, wash, and slice strawberries. Wash and pat the blueberries dry.

4. Heat some oil in a pan and bake small pancakes with 1 teaspoon of dough each over medium heat.

5. Serve the skewers, skewer a blueberry, then a strawberry slice, a pancake, a chocolate banana, and a pancake.

Nutrition:

- Calories 110
- Carbs 25g
- Fat 1g
- Protein 6g

Tomato and Zucchini Salad with Feta

Preparation Time: 0 minutes
Cooking Time: 20 minutes
Servings: 4

INGREDIENTS:

- 2 zucchinis
- 4 tbsp. olive oil
- Salt
- Pepper
- 400g tomatoes
- 200g cherry tomatoes
- 3 spring onions
- 1 bunch basil (20g)
- 2 tbsp. apple cider vinegar
- 100g feta (45% fat in dry matter)

DIRECTIONS:

1. Clean, wash, and cut zucchini. Heat 1 tablespoon of oil in a pan, fry the zucchini in it over medium heat for 5 minutes. Season with salt and pepper.

2. Clean, wash, and chop tomatoes. Wash and halve cherry tomatoes. Wash the spring onions and cut them into rings. Wash the basil, shake dry and pick the leaves.

3. Mix zucchini, tomatoes, cherry tomatoes, and basil. Add the remaining oil and apple cider vinegar, mix, and season with salt and pepper. Crumble the feta. Serve the salad sprinkled with feta.

NUTRITION:

- Calories 230 Cal
- Carbs 24g
- Fat 12g
- Protein 8g

Sirtfood Truffle Bites

Preparation Time: 1 hour
Cooking Time: 0 min
Servings: 15-20 pcs

INGREDIENTS:

- 1 cup walnuts
- ¾ cup of Medjool dates, pitted
- ½ cup of dark chocolate broken into pieces; or cocoa nibs
- 2 heaping tablespoons of cacao powder
- ½ cup of dried coconut
- 1 tbsp. ground turmeric
- 1 tbsp. extra virgin olive oil or coconut oil (preferred)
- 1 tsp. vanilla extract, or a vanilla pod, scraped
- 1 dash of cayenne pepper
- 1 dash sea salt (up to 1/8 teaspoon)
- 2 tbsp. water if needed

DIRECTIONS:

1. Pulse in a food processor the walnuts and chocolate until finely pulverized. Gently blend solid ingredients next and the vanilla. Make a dough. Make rolled balls out of the dough. Add water a few drops at a time only if it is necessary. Do not use too much water, or you will have to go and add more of the other ingredients to compensate. Refrigerate. Store for up to a week. Take them with you to work or when traveling for a quick pick-me-up as well as to quell a sweet tooth.

NUTRITION:

- Calories 256
- Fats 15

SPICY KALE CHIPS

Preparation Time: 2 hours 15 minutes
Cooking Time: 15 minutes
Servings: 1

INGREDIENTS:

- 1 large head of curly kale, wash, dry, and pulled from stem 1 tbsp. extra virgin olive oil
- Minced parsley
- Lemon juice
- Cayenne pepper (just a pinch)
- Dash of soy sauce

DIRECTIONS:

1. In a large bowl, rip the kale from the stem into palm-sized pieces. Sprinkle the minced parsley, olive oil, soy sauce, a squeeze of the lemon juice, and a very small pinch of the cayenne powder. Toss with a set of tongs or salad forks, and make sure to coat all of the leaves.

2. If you have a dehydrator, turn it on to 118 F, spread out the kale on a dehydrator sheet, and leave it there for about 2 hours.

3. If you are cooking them, place parchment paper on top of a cookie sheet, lay the bed of kale, and separate it a bit to make sure the kale is evenly toasted. Cook for 10-15 minutes maximum at 250F.

NUTRITION:

- Calories: 345
- Fats: 11

BANANA & GINGER SNAP

Preparation Time: 30 minutes
Cooking Time: 0 minutes
Servings: 1

INGREDIENTS:

- 2.5cm (1 inch) chunk of fresh ginger, peeled
- 1 banana
- 1 large carrot
- 1 apple, cored
- ½ stick of celery
- ¼ level teaspoon turmeric powder

DIRECTIONS:

1. Place all the ingredients into a blender with just enough water to cover them. Process until smooth

NUTRITION:

- Calories: 324
- Fats: 8

Chocolate, Strawberry & Coconut Crush

Preparation Time: 30 minutes
Cooking Time: 0 minutes
Servings: 1

INGREDIENTS:

- 100mls (3½fl oz) coconut milk
- 100g (3½oz) strawberries
- 1 banana
- 1 tablespoon 100% cocoa powder or cacao nibs
- 1 teaspoon matcha powder

DIRECTIONS:

1. Toss all of the ingredients into a blender and process them to a creamy consistency. Add a little extra water if you need to thin it a little.

NUTRITION:

- Calories: 289
- Fats: 16

CHOCOLATE BERRY BLEND

Preparation Time: 30 minutes
Cooking Time: 0 minutes
Servings: 1

INGREDIENTS:

- 50g (2oz) kale
- 50g (2oz) blueberries
- 50g (2oz) strawberries
- 1 banana
- 1 tablespoon 100% cocoa powder or cacao nibs
- 200mls (7fl oz) unsweetened soya milk

DIRECTIONS:

1. Place all of the ingredients into a blender with enough water to cover them and process until smooth.

NUTRITION:

- Calories: 256
- Fats: 9

Sweet and Savory Guacamole

Preparation Time: 20 minutes
Cooking Time: 0 minutes
Servings: 2

INGREDIENTS:

- 2 large avocados, pitted and scooped
- 2 Medjool dates, pitted and chopped into small pieces
- ½ cup cherry tomatoes cut into halves
- 5 sprigs of parsley, chopped
- ¼ cup of arugula, chopped
- 5 sticks of celery, washed, cut into sticks for dipping
- Juice from ¼ lime
- Dash of sea salt

DIRECTIONS:

1. Mash the avocado in a bowl, sprinkle salt, and squeeze of the lime juice. Fold in the tomatoes, dates, herbs, and greens. Scoop with celery sticks, and enjoy!

NUTRITION:

- Calories: 276
- Fats: 14

THAI NUT MIX

Preparation Time: 30 minutes
Cooking Time: 20 minutes
Servings: 1

INGREDIENTS:

- ½ cup walnuts
- ½ cup coconut flakes
- ½ tsp. soy sauce
- 1 tsp. honey
- 1 pinch of cayenne pepper
- 1 dash of lime juice

DIRECTIONS:

1. Add the above ingredients to a bowl, toss the nuts to coat, and place on a baking sheet, lined with parchment paper. Cook at 250 F for 15-20 minutes, checking as not to burn, but lightly toasted.

2. Remove from the oven. Cool first before eating.

NUTRITION:

- Calories: 322
- Fats: 12

Berry Yogurt Freeze

Preparation Time: 1 hour 30 minutes
Cooking Time: 0 minutes
Servings: 2

Ingredients:

- 2 cups plain yogurt (Greek, soy or coconut)
- ½ cup sliced strawberries
- ½ cup blackberries
- 1 tsp. honey (warmed) ½ tsp. chocolate powder

Directions:

1. Blend all of the above ingredients until creamy in a bowl. Place into two glass or in metal bowls that are freezer-safe, and put into the freezer for 1 hour, remove and thaw just slightly so that it is soft enough to eat with a spoon, makes two servings.

Nutrition:

- Calories: 289
- Fats: 16

BLUEBERRY AND COCONUT ROLLS

Preparation Time: 0 minutes
Cooking Time: 55 minutes
Servings: 4

INGREDIENTS

- 150g whole meal flour
- 150g spelled flour
- 1½ tsp. baking powder
- 1 pinch salt
- 50g raw cane sugar
- 4 tbsp. rapeseed oil
- 250g low-fat quark
- 1 egg
- 5 tbsp. milk (3.5% fat)
- 120g blueberries
- 4 tbsp. grated coconut

DIRECTIONS:

1. Put the flour with baking powder and salt in a bowl. Add sugar and mix. Add rapeseed oil, curd cheese, egg and 4 tablespoons of milk and use a hand mixer for kneading into a smooth dough.

2. Wash the blueberries, pat dry and fold in together with the grated coconut under the dough.

3. Line a baking sheet with parchment paper. Form 9 round rolls with floured hands and place them on the baking sheet. Brush the blueberry and coconut buns with the remaining milk and bake in a preheated oven at 200 ° C (fan oven 180 ° C; gas: setting 3) for 12–15 minutes.

NUTRITION:

- Calories: 140 Cal
- Carbs: 22g
- Fat: 5g
- Protein: 2g

Brain Food Cookies

Preparation Time: 0 minutes
Cooking Time: 52 minutes
Servings: 4

INGREDIENTS

- 150g spelled flour type 1050
- 1 tsp. baking powder
- 100g whole cane sugar
- 1 pinch salt
- 120g room temperature butter
- 3 ripe bananas
- 1 egg
- 150g pithy oatmeal
- 60g donated almonds
- 1 tbsp. cocoa nibs
- 2 tbsp. chocolate drop (made from dark chocolate; 15g)

DIRECTIONS:

1. Mix the flour with the baking powder, sugar and 1 pinch of salt. Add the butter in pieces and mix. Peel the bananas, mash them with a fork and add them to the dough together with the egg and stir well with a hand mixer. Fold in the oatmeal, almonds, cocoa nibs and half of the chocolate drops.

2. Line a baking sheet with parchment paper. Place the dough on the baking sheet with a tablespoon, leaving enough space between the cookies. Sprinkle with the remaining chocolate drops and bake in a preheated oven at 200 ° C (fan oven 180 ° C; gas: setting 3) for 10–15 minutes. Then let it cool down on a wire rack.

NUTRITION:

- Calories: 170 Cal
- Carbs: 8g
- Fat: 14g
- Protein: 6g

Conclusion

Thank you for making it to the end. Sirtfoods are the pioneering strategies to enact Sirtuin qualities in an ideal manner. These are magnificent nourishments that are especially wealthy in normal regular synthetic concoctions, called polyphenols, that can enact sirtuin qualities by actuating them. Basically, they imitate the impacts of fasting and practice and give astounding advantages by helping the body better control glucose, consume fat, form muscle, and improve wellbeing and memory.

Since plants are fixed, they have built up a propelled pressure reaction framework and produce polyphenols to adjust to the difficulties of their condition. At the point when we devour these plants, we likewise expend these polyphenolic supplements. Its impact is significant: they initiate our own natural pressure responses.

While all plants have pressure reaction frameworks, just a couple have advanced to deliver critical measures of the polyphenols that actuate sirtuin. These plants are grimy food. Their disclosure implies that rather than severe fasting programs or extreme exercise programs, there is presently a progressive better approach to actuate sirtuin qualities: an eating regimen rich in sirt. Best of all, diet is putting food on your plate and not getting more fit.

There is expanding proof that sirtuin activators have a few medical advantages, reinforce muscles, and smother hunger. These incorporate better memory, better control of the body's glucose levels, and disposal of harm brought about by free extreme atoms that amass in cells and can prompt malignant growth and different maladies.

"There are numerous perceptions about the useful impacts of utilizing sirtuin and food activators to decrease the danger of incessant infection," Professor Frank Hu, a nutritionist and disease transmission specialist at Harvard University, said in an ongoing report. Article in the magazine about dietary turns of events. A smart food diet is particularly appropriate as an enemy of the maturing diet.

In spite of the fact that sirtuin activators are available all through the plant realm, just particular sorts of products of the soil are sufficiently enormous to be considered Sirtuine nourishments. Models are green tea, cocoa powder, and turmeric with Indian flavors, cabbage, onion, and parsley.

Numerous foods are grown from the ground in plain view in grocery stores; for example, tomatoes, avocados, bananas, lettuce, kiwis, carrots, and cucumbers, really contain modest quantities of sirtuin activators. Nonetheless, this doesn't imply that it does not merit eating, as they offer numerous different advantages.

The beneficial thing about a sirt diet is that it is substantially more adaptable than different eating regimens. You can just eat well and include grimy food. Or then again, you could have gotten them. On the off chance that you include filthy food, a 5: 2 eating regimen can include more calories on low-calorie days.

An eminent finding from a sirt diet study is that members lost noteworthy load without losing muscle. Indeed, it was regular for members to really manufacture muscles, bringing about a clearer, firmer appearance. It is acceptable with sirt food. They enact fat consumption. However, they additionally advance muscle development, support, and fix. This is a conspicuous difference to different eating regimens where weight reduction, for the most part, results from both fat and muscle, with muscle misfortune easing back your digestion and making you bound to put on weight.

CONCLUSION

CPSIA information can be obtained
at www.ICGtesting.com
Printed in the USA
BVHW062327220321
003180BV00003D/623